DIABETIC

COOKBOOK FOR

BEGINNERS

Learn How To Cook Healthy Meals That Will Help Reverse Type 1 And Type 2 Diabetes

TINA TOWNSEND

original author of this work can be in any fashion deemed liable for any hardship or damages that may befall them after undertaking information described herein.

Additionally, the information in the following pages is intended only for informational purposes and should thus be thought of as universal. As befitting its nature, it is presented without assurance regarding its prolonged validity or interim quality. Trademarks that are mentioned are done without written consent and can in no way be considered an endorsement from the trademark holder.

TABLE OF CONTENTS

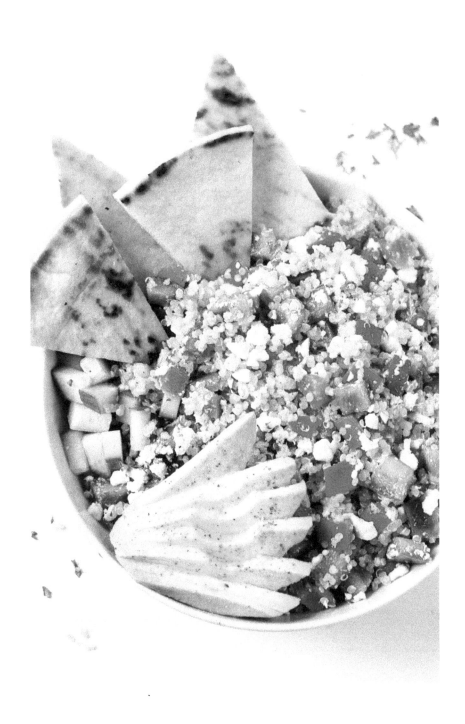

DIABETIC DATE DAINTIES

2 eggs

1 1/2 tsp. liquid sweetener

1 1/2 tsp. baking powder

1/3 c. dates, chopped

1/4 c. flour 1/2

c. nuts

1 1/2 c. bread crumbs

Beat eggs, sweetener and baking powder. Add dates, flour and nuts. Stir in bread crumbs. Chill, then measure by teaspoon on a greased cookie sheet. Bake at 375 degrees for 12 minutes.

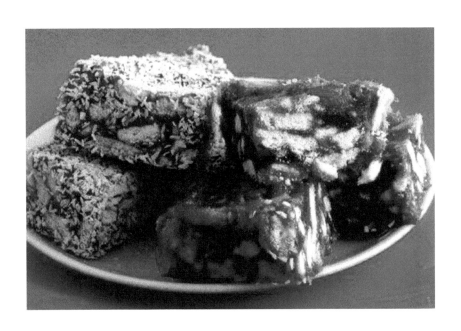

SUGAR - FREE CRANBERRY RELISH

2 c. cranberries

2 apples

1 c. orange juice

Grind together the cranberries and apples, using a sweet apple. (May also use blender). Add orange juice, chopped nuts and sweetener to taste. Refrigerate several hours before using.

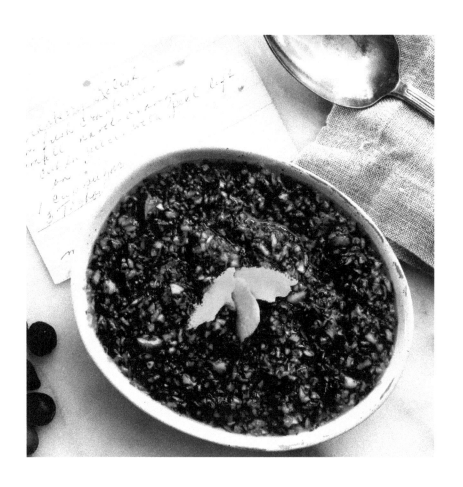

IT COULD BE A SNICKERS BAR

12 oz. soft diet ice cream

1 c. diet Cool Whip

1/4 c. chunky peanut butter

1 pkg. sugar free butterscotch pudding

(dry) 3 oz. Grape Nuts cereal

Mix first 4 ingredients in mixer, then stir in cereal. Pour into 8-inch square pan. Cover and freeze. Makes 4 servings.

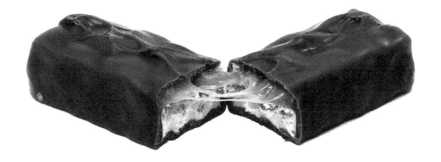

BAKED CHICKEN FOR ONE

1 (3 oz.) chicken breast, boned & skinned

2 tbsp. (any brand) bottled diet Italian dressing

Marinate chicken in dressing overnight in covered casserole. Bake for one hour at 350 degrees. No additional seasonings are necessary.

Will be very tender and juicy.

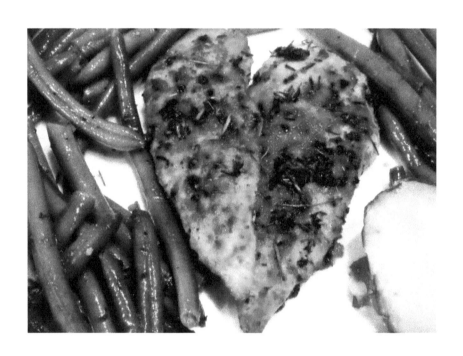

CHOCOLATE CHIP COOKIES

1/4 c. margarine

1 tbsp. granulated fructose

1 egg

1 tsp. vanilla extract

3/4 c. flour

1/4 tsp. salt

1/2 c. mini semi-sweet chocolate chips

Cream together margarine and fructose, beat in egg, water and vanilla. Combine flour, baking soda and salt in sifter. Sift dry ingredients into creamed mixture, stirring to blend thoroughly. Stir in chocolate chips. Drop by teaspoonsful onto lightly greased cookie sheet about 2 inches apart. Bake at 375 degrees for 8 to 10 minutes. Makes 30 cookies.

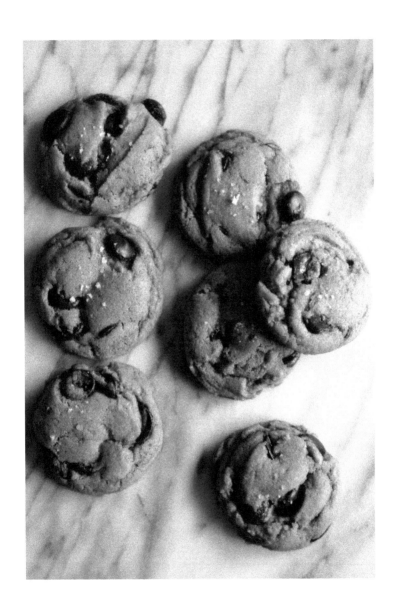

ORANGE RICE

1 c. rice, uncooked 1
c. water

1 c. orange juice

1 tsp. reduced calorie margarine
Dash of salt

1 tbsp. orange rind, freshly grated
1/2 c. fresh orange sections, seeded

In a 2-quart microwave safe casserole, combine the rice, water, orange juice, margarine and salt. Cover, microwave on High for 5 minutes. Stir in the orange rind. Turn the bowl 1/4 turn. Microwave on High for an additional 10 minutes, turning the bowl after 5 minutes. Do not uncover the bowl. Allow to set covered for an additional 10 minutes or until all of the liquids have been absorbed. Immediately before serving, fluff with a fork, add orange sections and mix gently.

Serve with pride. Makes about 6 (100 calories) servings.

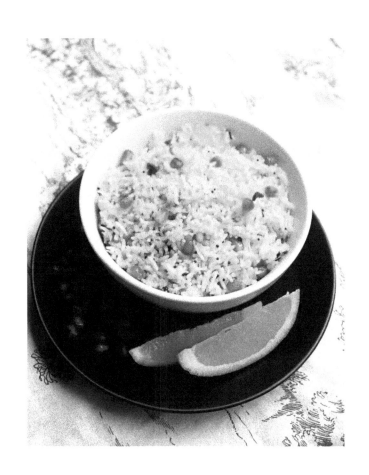

BLACK BOTTOM PIE

GRAHAM CRACKER CRUST:

1 1/4 c. graham cracker crumbs

1/2 c. diet margarine

FILLING

1 envelope unflavored gelatine

3/4 c. part skim ricotta cheese

12 packets sweetener

1 packet low calorie whipped topping
mix 1 1/2 c. skim milk

1 tbsp. vanilla extract

1/4 c. cocoa

Combine crumbs with diet margarine by cutting in softened margarine until mixture resembles coarse crumbs. Press firmly in bottom and sides of 8- or 9-inch pie pan. Bake in preheated 350-degree oven for 8 to 10 minutes. Cool. In small saucepan, sprinkle gelatine over 1/2 cup skim milk. Let stand one minute.

Heat, stirring constantly until gelatine dissolves. In blender or food processor, blend ricotta until smooth and add gelatine mixture, remaining 1 cup milk and vanilla. Continue blending until completely smooth. Remove half the mixture, set aside. To mixture still in blender, add 6 packs sugar substitute and cocoa. Blend thoroughly. Pour blender mixture into crust, chill for 30 minutes or until partially set. At the same time, chill remaining mixture for 30 minutes.

Prepare whipped topping mix according to package directions gradually adding remaining 6 packets sugar substitute. Whisk into reserved, chilled mixture until blended smoothly. Spoon over chocolate layer; chill until set. Garnish with dusting of cocoa. Makes one (8 or 9 inch) pie or 8 servings.

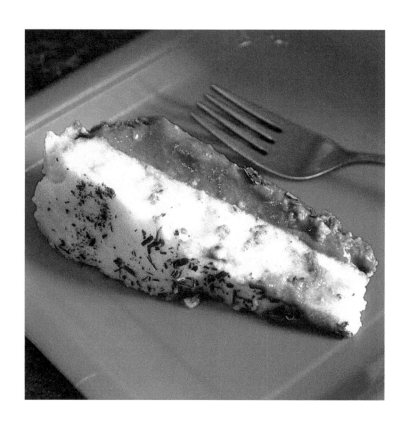

CHICKEN BREASTS WITH CARROT AND ZUCCHINI STUFFING

2 small (whole) skinless, boneless chicken breasts 1 c. carrots, shredded (about 2 sm.)

1 c. zucchini, shredded (about 1 med.)

1 tsp. salt

1/4 tsp. poultry seasoning

1 envelope chicken flavoured bouillon 1/4 c. water

In medium bowl, combine carrots, zucchini, salt and poultry seasoning. Spoon about 1/2 cup mixture into each pocket (each breast should open similar to a butterfly); secure with toothpicks. In place chicken in a Med size skillet, sprinkle with bouillon.

Add water to skillet and cook over medium high heat, heat to boiling. Reduce heat to low; cover and simmer about 40 minutes or until chicken is fork tender. Remove toothpicks. Makes 4 servings, 180 calories per serving.

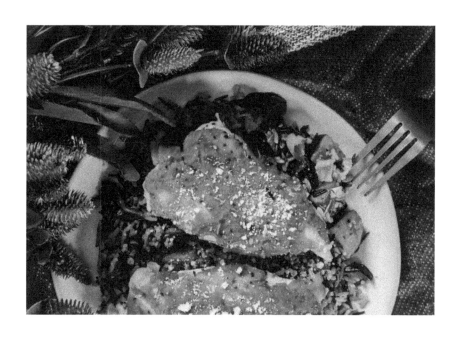

SUGARLESS CAKE

1 c. dates, chopped 1

c. prunes, chopped 1

c. raisins

1 c. cold water

1 stick margarine, melted

2 eggs

1 tsp. baking soda 1/4

tsp. salt

1 c. plain flour

1 c. nuts, chopped

1/4 tsp. cinnamon

1/4 tsp. nutmeg

1 tsp. vanilla

Boil dates and prunes in the one cup of water for 3 minutes; add margarine and raisins and let cool. Mix flour, soda, salt, eggs, nuts, spices and vanilla. Add to fruit mixture. Stir to blend. Pour into baking dish. Bake at 350 degrees for 25 to 30 minutes.

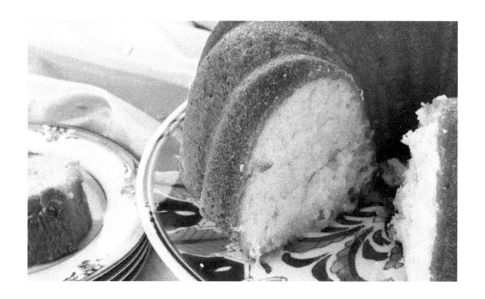

DIABETIC ORANGE SUNBEAMS

1 1/2 c. all-purpose flour

1 tsp. baking powder 1/4

tsp. salt

1/2 c. shortening 1/2

c. raisins

1 egg

2 tbsp. orange juice

2 tsp. grated orange rind 1

1/2 tsp. Sucaryl

Sift together flour, baking powder and salt. Cut in shortening until crumbly. Add all at once: raisins, eggs, orange juice, orange rind and Sucaryl. Mix well. Make into small balls; flatten on cookie sheet.

Bake 12 to 15 minutes at 375 degrees.

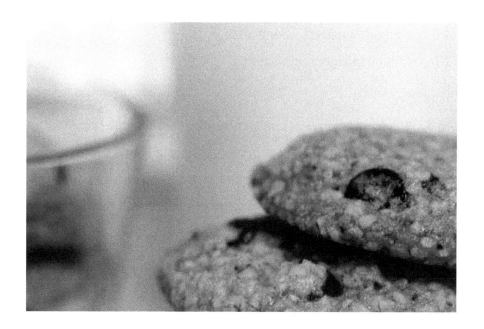

ALMOND BISCUIT RING

1/4 c. granulated brown sugar, replacement

2 tbsp. dietetic maple syrup

2 tsp. reduced calorie margarine

2 tsp. water

1/3 c. almonds, coarsely chopped

1 (8 oz.) tube refrigerator biscuits

In a 1 1/2-quart microwave safe casserole, combine the brown sugar replacement, maple syrup, margarine and water. Cover with a paper towel and microwave on high for one minute. Allow to sit, covered for one minute, then stir to mix in the melted margarine. Stir in the almonds. Cut each of the biscuits into four pieces.

Roll each piece into a ball. Dip each piece into the syrup mixture then place in a microwave safe ring mold. Arrange all coated balls uniformly around the ring mold. Pour any remaining syrup over the balls in the mold.

Microwave on medium (50% power) for 5 to 6 minutes, turning the mold 1/4 turn after each two minutes. Remove from oven and immediately cover with waxed paper. Allow to sit undisturbed 5 minutes; then turn out onto a serving dish. Divide into 10 servings. About 80 calories per serving.

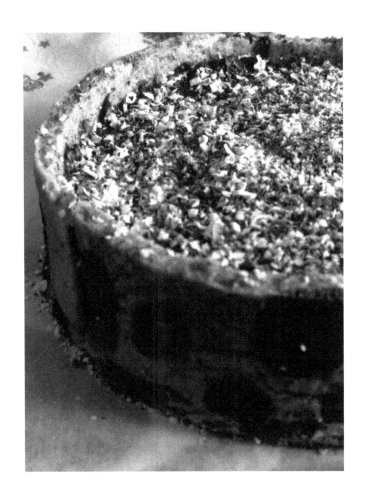

BANANA SPLIT PIE

1 graham cracker crust

1 (4 oz.) pkg. sugar free instant vanilla pudding
mix 2 c. low fat milk

2 bananas, sliced

1 (15 oz.) can crushed pineapple

1 c. Cool Whip

1 tsp. vanilla

1/2 c. pecans, chopped

Mix pudding with milk and beat until thick, pour into crust. Put
bananas over pudding. Squeeze pineapple to remove all juice.
Sprinkle on top of bananas. Cover with Cool Whip, sprinkle
pecans on top. Chill well.

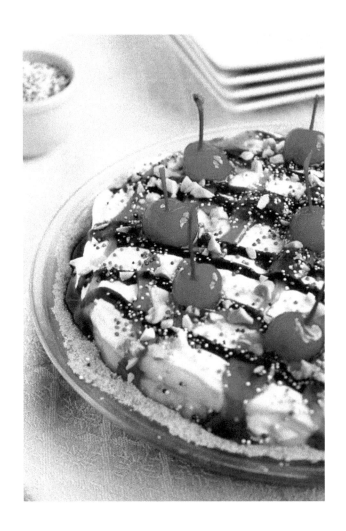

FRUIT DIP

1 c. plain yogurt 8
oz. light cream

8 packets Equal sugar 1
tsp. vanilla.

Mix all ingredients together.

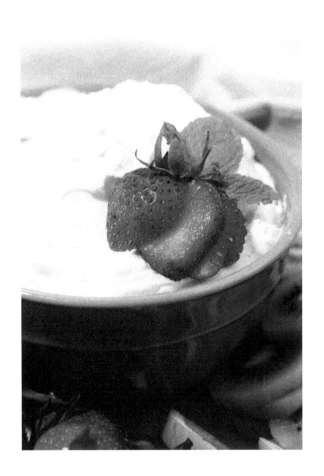

BROWNIE TORTE

1 1/2 c. chilled whipping
cream 3 tbsp. Fruit Sweet or to
taste 1 tsp. vanilla

Prepare Fudge Sweet Brownies (see recipe below). Whip cream,
Fruit Sweet and vanilla and use as filling and topping for layers of
brownies. Low Fat Substitute: About 3 cups frozen whipped
topping, thawed.

Substitute your favourite flavouring for the vanilla, such as 1
tablespoon instant coffee or 1 tablespoon concentrated orange juice.

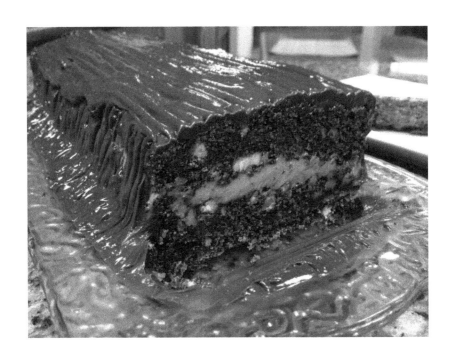

FUDGE SWEET BROWNIES

2/3 c. flour

1/2 tsp. baking powder 2
eggs, beaten well

1/2 c. melted butter or oil 1/2
c. Fudge Sweet, softened 1/2
c. Fruit Sweet

1 tsp. vanilla

1/2 c. walnuts, chopped

Sift flour and baking powder; set aside. Blend the eggs, butter or oil, Fudge Sweet, Fruit Sweet and vanilla. Add the flour mixture and blend thoroughly. Add walnuts. Pour mixture into greased and floured 8"x8" baking pan. Bake at 350 degrees for about 15 minutes, until cake springs back at a light touch. Doubled recipe will fit into double size cookie pan.

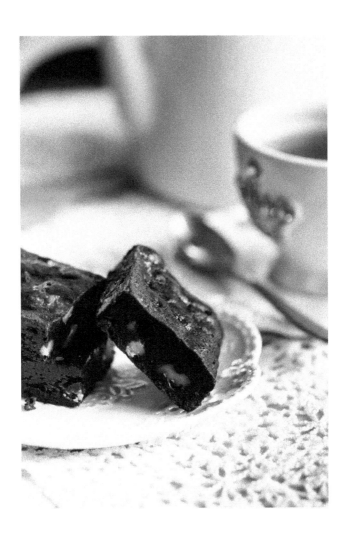

FROZEN APRICOT MOUSSE

1 c. apricot apple butter

1/2 c. whipping cream 2

egg whites

2 tbsp. Fruit Sweet

Beat egg whites until stiff but not dry. Fold into the apricot apple butter. Whip the cream until stiff, adding the Fruit Sweet. Fold the whipped cream into the apricot mixture. Freeze.

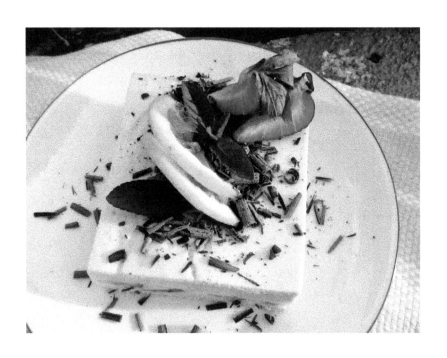

FRUIT LEATHER

Place a sheet of plastic wrap in the bottom of a cookie sheet. Smooth a thin layer of fruit butter with the edge of a pancake turner. Place in the oven to dry at the lowest heat, about 120, for about 2 hours, or until dry, then remove and cool. Peel off and roll in plastic wrap. For variety, sprinkle with finely chopped walnuts before drying.

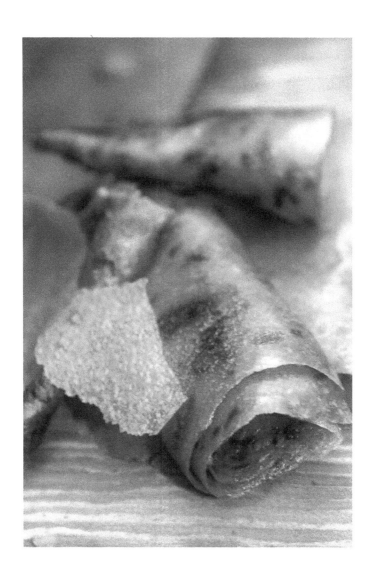

FRUIT SALAD TOPPING

1 1/2 c. milk (skim or 1%)

1 (3 oz.) sugar free vanilla pudding

Add: 2 tbsp. frozen orange juice
concentrate 1 tsp. grated orange peel (opt.)

Can be served as a side dish with mixed fruit (fresh) or mix fruit
and topping in bowl.

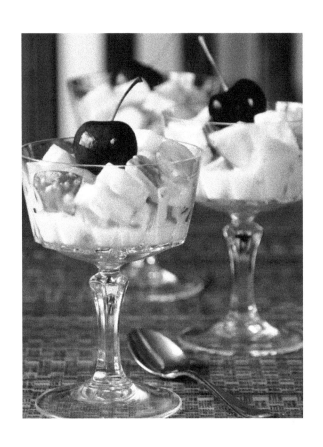

RASPBERRY MOUSSE

2/3 c. Strawberry Fanciful

1/8 tsp. cream of tartar

2 egg whites

1/2 c. whipping cream

Add cream of tartar to egg whites, beat until stiff, but not dry.
Fold into Strawberry Fanciful. Fold the whipped cream into the
fruit mixture. Chill before serving or freeze for frozen mousse.
For flavour variation try: Strawberry, blueberry, orange
pineapple, pineapple berry or peach.

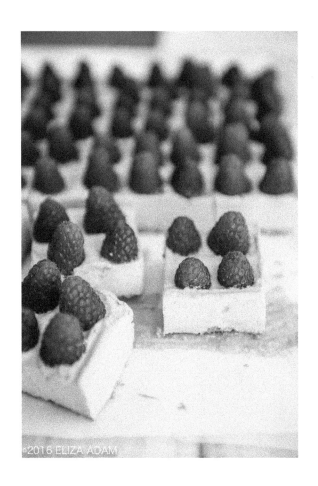

GOLDEN CARROT PIE

2 eggs

1/4 tsp. ground cinnamon

Pinch salt

1/2 c. Fruit Sweet 9"

pie shell

Dash ground nutmeg

1/8 tsp. ground ginger

1 c. cooked carrots, riced or mashed

1/2 c. heavy cream

Beat the eggs, nutmeg, cinnamon, ginger and salt until
thoroughly blended. Add the carrots and stir well. Pour in the
Fruit Sweet and cream and stir until completely blended. Pour
the filling into the pie shell and bake at 350 degrees for 35
minutes or until a knife inserted in the center comes clean. Serve
with whipped topping.

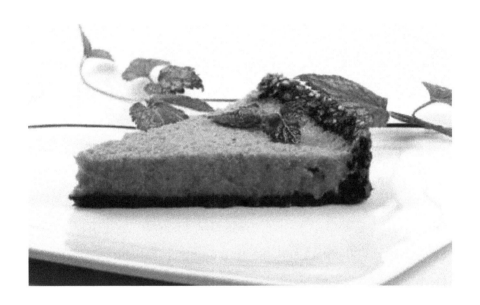

APPLESAUCE CAKE

2 eggs, well beaten 1

c. Apple Butter

1 1/2 c. flour

1/2 c. raisins

1/2 c. butter, melted

1/2 c. Fruit Sweet

1 1/2 tsp. baking soda

1/2 c. chopped walnuts

Combine the eggs, butter and apple butter. Sift the flour and bake soda. Add the walnuts and raisins to the flour mixture and blend. Add the flour mixture to the egg mixture alternately with the Fruit Sweet. Pour the batter into a greased tube pan and bake at 375 degrees for 30 to 35 minutes. Turn out and cool before serving. Serve with whipped cream.

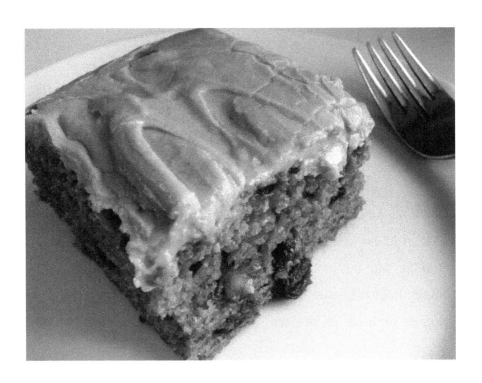

EASY CHOCOLATE GRAHAM TORTE

Line 13"x9"x2" pan with a layer of graham cracker squares. Prepare 1 large (6 oz.) package of instant sugar free chocolate pudding as directed on the package. Spread over graham cracker layer. Place in refrigerator to let set a little.

Layer another layer of graham cracker squares over the pudding. Prepare a second package of chocolate pudding as above and spread over graham crackers. *Refrigerate*. Torte may be topped with whipped cream or Dream Whip when served. This easy dessert is one that diabetics may enjoy.

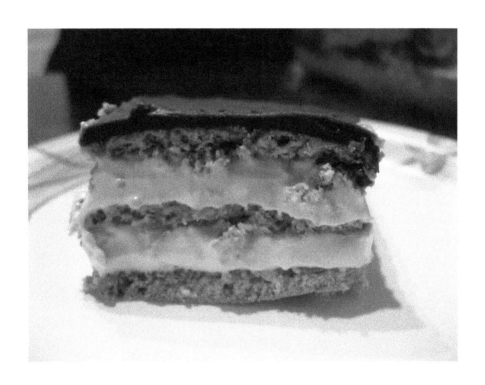

FANCIFUL FREEZE

4 ripe bananas, peeled 1/2
c. Raspberry Fanciful

Wrap bananas in plastic wrap and freeze overnight. Remove from freezer, break into 4 or 5 pieces and let stand at room temperature for about 10 minutes to slightly soften for the processor. Blend the bananas in a processor or blender until creamy. Add the Raspberry (or other flavour) Fanciful and blend briefly. This can be served immediately, or stored in the freezer. Serves 4.

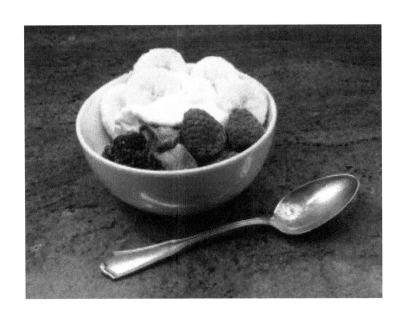

NO-SUGAR CUSTARD

6 egg yolks

1/4 c. Fruit Sweet
1/2 c. flour

2 c. milk

1 tsp. vanilla

1 tbsp. butter

In a medium bowl, beat egg yolks and Fruit Sweet until thick and pale. While continuing to beat, gradually sift in flour. Pour into a saucepan and place over low heat on the stove and gradually add milk and vanilla. Cook, stirring constantly, until mixture has thickened to a custard consistency, about 15 minutes. Remove from heat. Melt butter and pour over custard to prevent a skin from forming while it cools. Makes 3 cups.

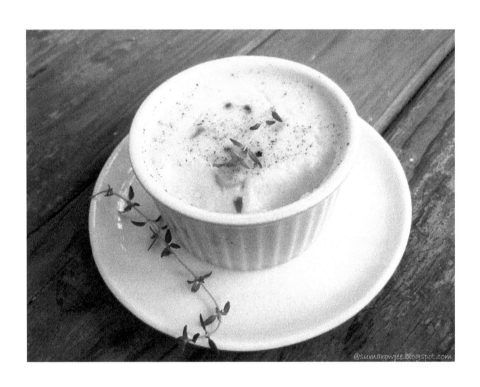

CHOCOLATE CAKE

2 eggs, beaten

1/2 c. butter, melted

1 c. strawberry apple butter

1 tsp. vanilla

5 tbsp. milk

3/4 c. Fudge Sweet Topping

5 tbsp. Fruit Sweet

2 c. flour

2 tsp. baking powder

Combine eggs, butter, strawberry apple butter and vanilla. Place the covered jar of Fudge Sweet into hot water to thin. Add the milk, Fudge Sweet and Fruit Sweet to the butter mixture. Sift the flour and baking soda together and blend with the wet mixture. Pour into two greased and floured 9" round tins or equivalent. Bake at 350 degrees for 40 minutes. Cool. Top with whipped cream.

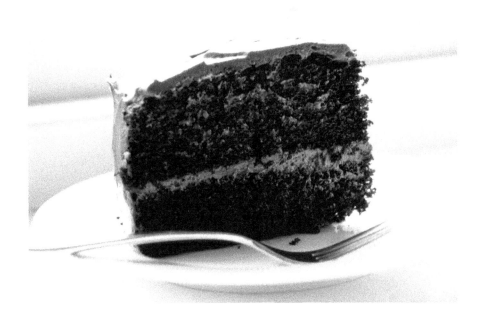

ORANGE MINCE CAKE

2 eggs, well beaten

1/3 c. Fruit Sweet 1

1/2 c. flour

1 1/2 tsp. baking powder

1/4 c. butter

1 c. Fruit Mincemeat

1 tsp. baking soda

Beat eggs, melt butter and add to Mincemeat and Fruit Sweet. Sift dry ingredients, add to mincemeat mix and blend. Spoon and smooth batter into oiled and floured 8" baking pan. Bake at 350 degrees for approximately 25 minutes. Top with Orange Cream Cheese Topping.

ORANGE CREAM CHEESE FROSTING

6 oz. cream cheese 2 tbsp. Fruit Sweet

2 tbsp. concentrated orange juice

Blend all ingredients together. Use on Orange Mince Cake.

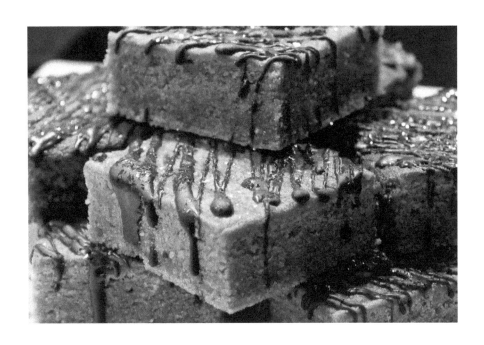

LO-CAL CHEESE CAKE

12 oz. low fat Ricotta cheese

4 eggs, separated

3/4 c. Fruit Sweet

Grated peel of 1 lemon

3 graham crackers, finely crushed

12 oz. low fat cottage cheese

2/3 c. non instant milk powder

5 tbsp. lemon juice or to taste 2

tsp. pure vanilla

Butter or oleo for pan

Put cheese in process with egg yolks and Fruit Sweet and blend. Add milk, powder and process until smooth. Add vanilla, lemon juice and peel to cheese mixture. Blend until smooth. Beat egg whites until frothy, then add to the processor and blend for about 2 seconds, until mixed. Butter the bottom and 1/2 way up the sides of a 9" springform pan.

Pour the graham cracker crumbs into the pan and shake until buttered area is coated. Leave any extra on the bottom. Pour cheesecake mixture into pan and bake at 350 degrees with a pan of water in the oven to prevent drying.　　Bake for 45 minutes or until inserted knife emerges clean. Cool. May serve with Wax Orchards All Fruit Fanciful preserve of your choice. *Variations: All cottage or all ricotta cheese may be used. For standard cream cheese cake, substitute 24 ounces cream cheese, 3 eggs, 1/2 cup powdered milk and 2/3 cup Fruit Sweet. Adjust lemon.*

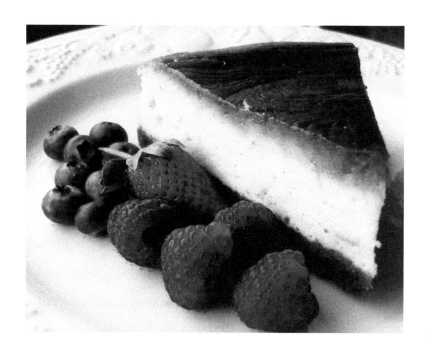

APRICOT PINEAPPLE CAKE

2 eggs, beaten

3/4 c. Apricot Apple Butter

1/2 c. dried apricots, chopped fine

2 tsp. baking soda

1/2 c. butter, melted

1/2 c. drained, crushed pineapple

2 c. flour

1/2 c. Fruit Sweet

Combine the eggs, butter, Apricot Apple Butter, pineapple and dried apricots until thoroughly blended. Mix the flour and baking soda together, then combine with the egg mixture alternately with the Fruit Sweet. Mix until the batter is smooth. Bake in a 9"x12" greased and floured pan at 340 degrees for 40 minutes or until cake springs back when pressed lightly. Remove the cake from the oven. Cool, turn out and cool completely. Flavour is usually better the next day.

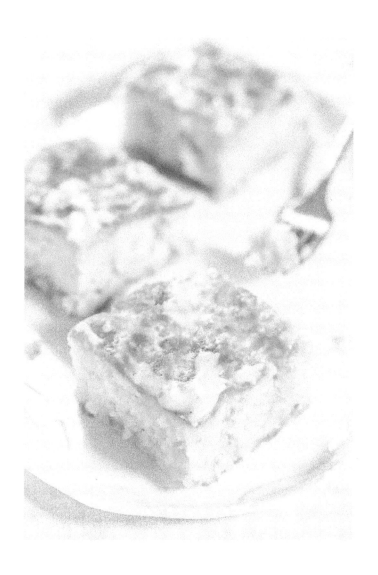

REFRIGERATOR BRAN MUFFINS

1 1/2 c. apple juice 1

c. butter, melted 4

well beaten eggs 4

c. buttermilk

5 tsp. baking soda

2 c. processed Bran Buds

1 c. Fruit Sweet

4 c. ready to eat bran cereal 5

c. flour

1 tsp. salt

Pour the juice into a medium saucepan and bring to a boil over high heat. Remove, pour in the Bran Buds and stir well. Let the mixture stand for several minutes. Combine the butter, Fruit Sweet and eggs and beat well. Then stir in the bran cereal. Pour in the buttermilk and stir well, then add the flour, baking soda and salt. Beat the batter until it is thoroughly blended.

Add the juice and Bran Buds and stir the batter until well blended. Drop several teaspoonfuls of batter into each greased muffin cup. Bake at 400 degrees for 15 minutes or until the center of each muffin is done. The batter can be stored in the refrigerator for up to 6 weeks and used as needed. Fruit and nuts, such as raisins, cranberries, bananas and walnuts, can be finely chopped, tossed with a little flour can also be used to add a little variety.

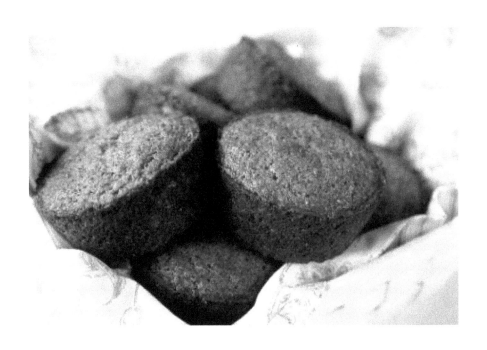

BUTTER POUNDCAKE

2 eggs, separated

6 tbsp. butter, softened 2

tsp. vanilla

2 tsp. baking powder

4 tbsp. whipping cream

3/4 c. Fruit Sweet

1 3/4 c. sifted cake flour

1 tsp. baking soda

Beat the egg yolks well. Add cream, butter, Fruit Sweet and vanilla and beat to blend well. Set aside. Sift the flour, baking powder and baking soda together and set aside in a small bowl. In a medium size bowl, slowly blend the flour mixture and the liquid mixture in small amounts at a time until well mixed. Beat until smooth.

In a separate bowl, beat egg whites until stiff but not dry. Stir a third of the whites into the batter and then gently fold in the remainder.

Spoon into a greased and floured 9" pan. Bake in a preheated 350-degree oven for 25 to 35 minutes or until an inserted straw or toothpick comes out dry. Cool for about 5 minutes before turning out onto rack.

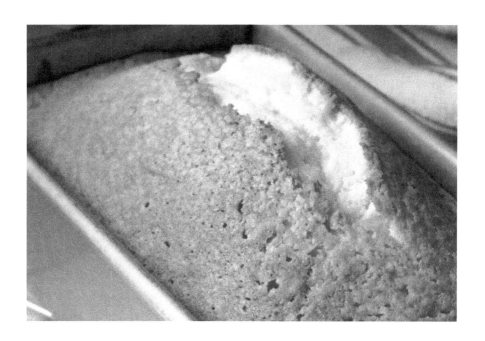

TORTE AU CHOCOLA

1 3/4 c. cake flour, sifted

1/43 tsp. salt

3 tsp. baking powder

1/2 tsp. cinnamon

4 eggs, separated

1/2 c. melted butter or oil

3/4 c. Fruit Sweet

3/4 c. Fudge Sweet 1

tsp. vanilla

1/2 c. milk

Sift dry ingredients together and set aside. Combine the butter or oil, Fruit Sweet, Fudge Sweet and vanilla. Add the yolks to the liquid mixture, blending one at a time. Add the flour mixture to the liquid mixture alternately with the milk. Whip the egg whites to stiff peaks and fold in gently but thoroughly. Bake at 350 degrees for 1/2 hour in 2 (9") round greased and floured tins. Test. Cake will spring back when lightly touched. _For a drier cake, bake until the cake draws away from the edge of the pan._ Cool.

FILLING

1 (8 oz.) pkg. cream cheese

3 tbsp. Fruit Sweet

1 tsp. vanilla

Blend together. Cream cheese may be warmed slightly to soften for blending. Fill cake, then frost with whipped cream sweetened to taste with Fruit Sweet, flavoured with vanilla or your favourite flavouring.

Drizzle melted Fruit Sweet around edge of cake. *optional - put thinly sliced strawberries on top.*

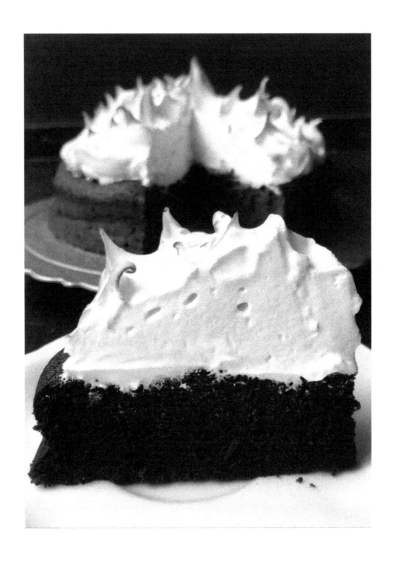

DIABETIC OATMEAL PEANUT BUTTER COOKIES

2/3 c. oatmeal 2
c. flour

1 tsp. lite salt
1/4 tsp. soda
2 tsp. baking powder
1/3 c. corn oil
2/3 c. salt free peanut butter
1/4 c. Eggbeaters and 1 egg 3
tbsp. skim milk

4 tbsp. liquid sweetener
2 tbsp. sugar substitute

Sift flour, salt, soda, and baking powder. Cream next 6 ingredients together add oatmeal, beat. Add flour mixture, stir until it forms a ball; roll into 1-inch balls. Place on ungreased cookie sheet. Press down with glass. Bake at 375 degrees for 10 minutes. approx. 35 calories per cookie.

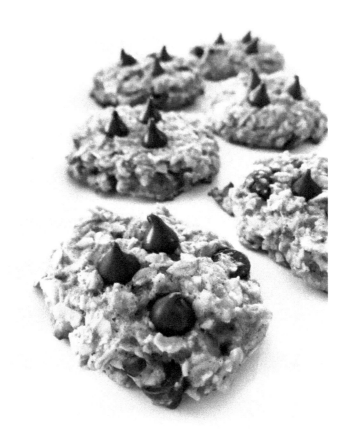

DIABETIC PEANUT BUTTER COOKIES

1 c. flour

1/2 c. creamy peanut butter 1
egg

1 tsp. vanilla
1/4 tsp. salt

1 1/2 tsp. baking powder
1/2 c. water

1 tbsp. liquid sweetener
1/2 c. salad oil

Mix all together in a large bowl. Shape into balls and place on
ungreased cookie sheet. Bake at 375 degrees for 12 to 15
minutes. (You may add a little more flour if desired.)

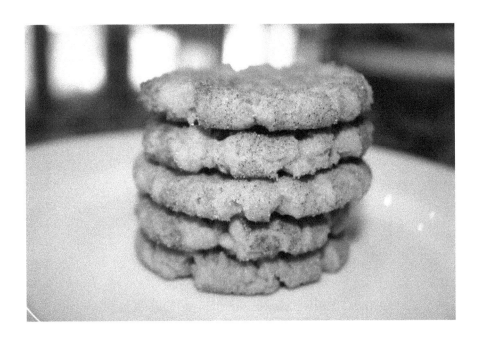

DIABETIC PEANUT BUTTER COOKIES

1/3 c. plain flour 1/4
tsp. baking soda

1/4 tsp. baking powder
Pinch of salt

2 tbsp. shortening
2 tbsp. peanut butter 1
tsp. Sweet 'n Low 1
egg, beaten

Mix and stir all ingredients in order (flour, baking soda, baking powder, salt, shortening, peanut butter and Sweet 'n Low). Add beaten egg and mix well. Drop by large teaspoon on greased cookie sheet. Bake at 350 degrees for 10 minutes.

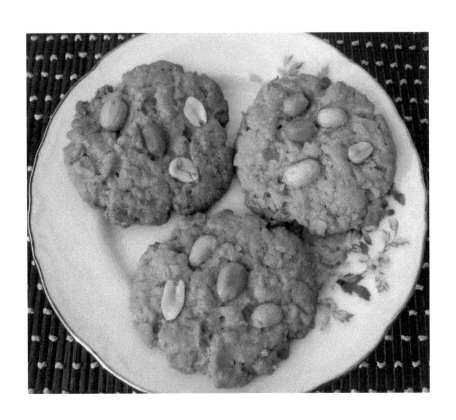

DIABETIC FUDGE

1 14 1/2 oz. evaporated milk

3 tbsp. cocoa

1/4 c. oleo

Liquid Sweetener to equal 1/2 c. sugar

1/4 tsp. salt

1 tsp. vanilla

2 1/2 c. graham cracker crumbs

1/4 c. nuts

Combine milk and cocoa in saucepan. Beat well. Add oleo, sweetener, salt. Bring to boil. Remove from heat. Stir in remaining ingredients except 1/4 cup graham crackers. Cool about 15 minutes. Divide mixture into 32 balls. Roll in remaining cracker crumbs and chill.

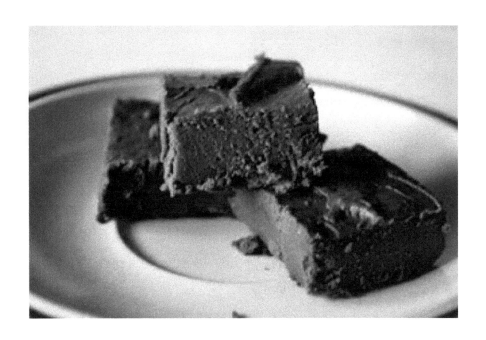

PINEAPPLE SHERBET (FOR DIABETICS)

1 (16 oz.) can crushed pineapple in pineapple
juice 1 tsp. unflavored gelatin (1/3 envelope)
2 tbsp. lemon juice nonnutritive sweetener equivalent to 1/2 cup
sugar 1/2 c. nonfat dry milk powder

At least 3 1/2 hours before serving: Drain pineapple, reserving
juice. In small saucepan, into 1/4 cup reserved pineapple juice,
sprinkle gelatine. Cook over low heat, stirring constantly until
gelatine is dissolved. Remove from heat; stir in 1/2 cup reserved
pineapple juice, lemon juice, crushed pineapple and non-nutritive
sweetener; cool.   In
small bowl with mixer at high speed, beat milk powder with 1/2
cup ice water until stiff peaks form; gently stir in gelatine mixture
until well combined. Pour into shallow pan; freeze 3 hours or until
firm. Makes 8 servings.

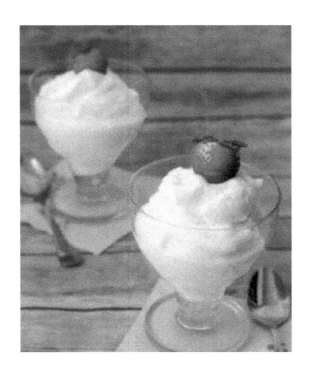

ORANGE SHERBET (FOR DIABETICS)

1 c. orange juice

1 tsp. unflavoured gelatine (1/3 envelope) 2 tbsp. lemon juice

1 tbsp. grated orange peel non-nutritive sweetener equal to 1/2 cup sugar

1/2 c. non-fat dry milk powder

Mix all ingredients together until well blended.

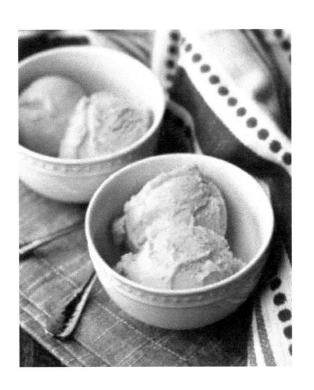

DIABETIC APPLE PIE

Pastry for 8-inch two crust pie

6 c. sliced tart apples

3/4 tsp. cinnamon or nutmeg

1 (12 oz.) can frozen Seneca apple
juice 2 tbsp. corn starch

Heat oven to 425 degrees. Put apples in pastry lined pan. Heat juice, corn starch and spice (optional). Let it boil until clear. Pour over apples. Cover with top crust. Bake 50 to 60 minutes.

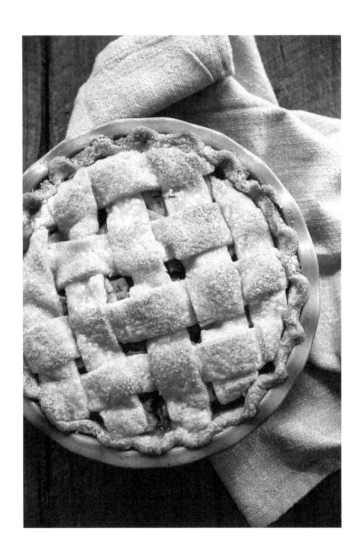

DIABETIC'S PUMPKIN PIE

1 baked, cooked 9-inch pie shell

2 sm. pkgs. sugar free instant vanilla pudding c. milk

1 c. canned pumpkin

1 tsp. pumpkin pie spice

1/4 tsp. nutmeg

1/4 tsp. ginger 1/2

tsp. cinnamon

Blend all ingredients in blender until smooth. Use plain canned pumpkin. Do not use canned pumpkin pie mixture. Pour into pie shell and chill until ready to serve.

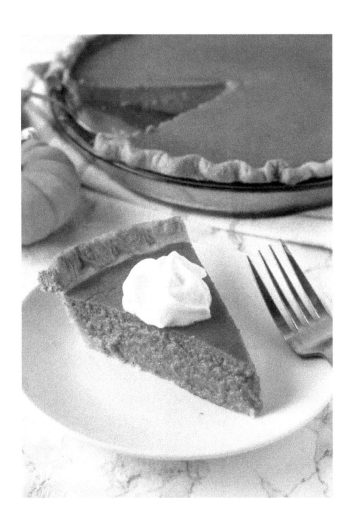

SUGAR-FREE DIABETIC CAKE

2 c. raisins

2 c. water

2 eggs, lightly beaten (you can use eggbeaters or egg whites) 1 tsp. vanilla extract

1/2 c. skim milk

2 c. unsweetened applesauce

3 tsp. Sweet & Low

1 tsp. cinnamon

1 tsp. nutmeg

1 tsp. salt

1 tsp. baking powder 2 c. all-purpose flour

1 c. chopped nuts (optional)

You may substitute the nuts with 1/2 cup mashed bananas for a uniquely different flavour, if so, mix banana with the wet ingredients. Preheat oven to 350 degrees. Cook raisins in water until all water is absorbed, about 30 minutes. Mix all the wet ingredients in one bowl and all the dry ingredients in a separate bowl. The nuts get added to the flour mixture then add the flour mixture to the liquid mixture. Fold in the raisins. Bake in loaf or bundt pan for 35 to 45 minutes or until toothpick inserted comes out clean.

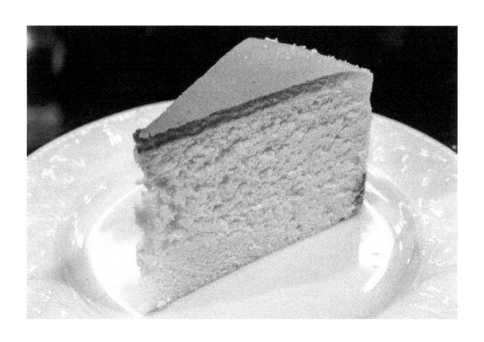

STRAWBERRY DIABETIC JAM

1 c. berries

3/4 c. sugar free strawberry pop 1
pkg. strawberry sugar free Jello 3
packets Equal

Mash the berries, add soda pop and cook 1 minute. Remove from heat and stir in Jello until dissolved. Stir in sweetener and pour in jars.

Seal and store in refrigerator. Yields about 1 1/4 cups. You may use other fruits such as raspberries, peaches or cherries.

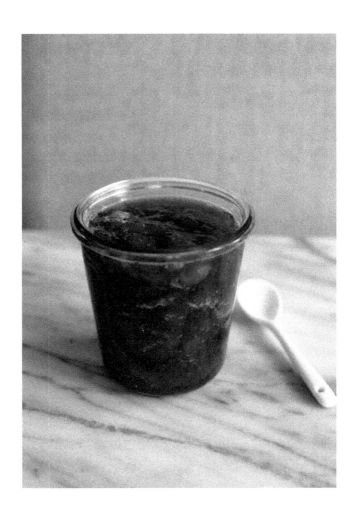

DIABETIC PUNCH

1 2-liter diet Sprite

1 (46 oz.) can chilled unsweetened pineapple
juice 1 pkg. blueberry Kool Aid with
NutraSweet

Chill all ingredients and pour in punch bowl and serve.

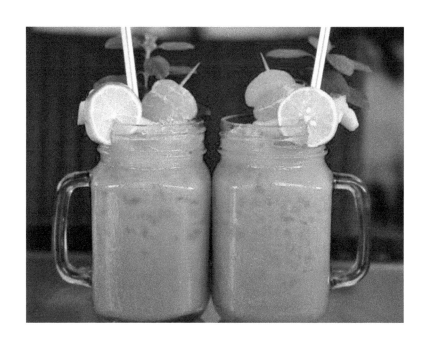

DIABETIC EGG NOG

1 1/2 c. milk

5 sucaryl tablets

4 eggs, beaten well 2
tsp. vanilla

Put all ingredients together and mix well.

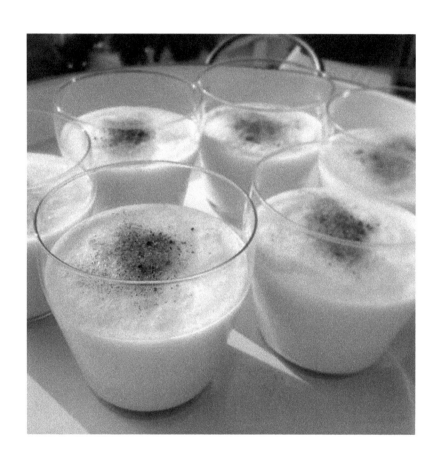

DIABETIC JELLY

1 qt. sugarless apple juice

4 tbsp. artificial sweetener (can add more)

4 tbsp. lemon juice

2 pkg. unflavoured gelatine

Mix ingredients and boil gently for 5 minutes. Cool and pour into containers. Store in refrigerator.

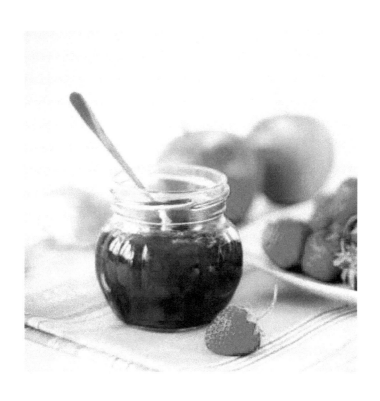

DIABETIC COOKIES

1 c. raisins

1 c. water

2 eggs, beaten

1 tsp. vanilla

1 c. flour

1/4 c. dates, chopped

1/2 c. shortening

3 tsp. sweetener

1 tsp. soda

Boil raisins, dates and water for 3 minutes. Add shortening and cool. Add eggs, then all remaining ingredients and mix well. Chill. Drop onto ungreased cookie sheet. Bake at 350 degrees for 10 to 12 minutes.

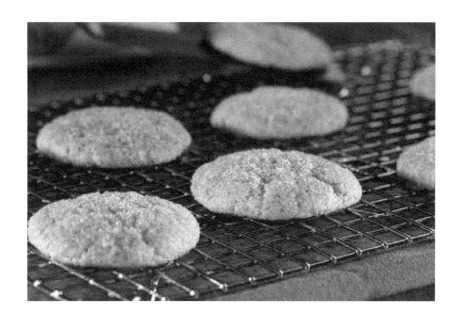

DIABETIC FRUIT COOKIES

1 c. flour

1 tsp. baking soda 1
c. water

1 c. dates, chopped
1/2 c. apples, peeled & chopped
3/4 c. raisins

1/2 c. margarine 1
c. quick oats

2 eggs, beaten (or eggbeaters)
1 tsp. vanilla
1 c. pecans, chopped

Sift flour and soda, set aside. Cook water, dates, apple and raisins; bring to a boil. Simmer 3 minutes. Remove from heat and add the margarine and stir. Cool mixture and then add eggs, oatmeal and the dry ingredients; add the vanilla and nuts. Cover and refrigerate overnight. Drop on cookie sheets 2 inches apart. Bake in 350-degree oven for about 24 minutes. Store in the refrigerator in air tight container. May also add 1 tsp. cinnamon to dry ingredients if desired.

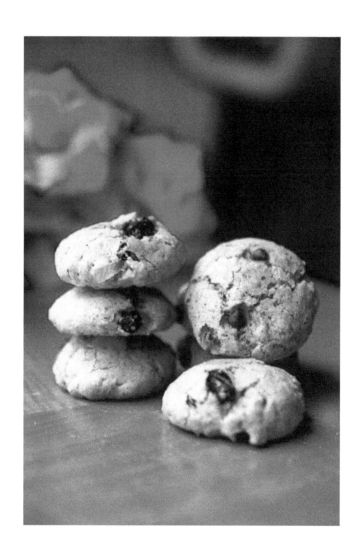

BAKE DIABETIC FRUIT CAKE

1 lb. graham crackers, crushed (reserve 3 double crackers)

1/2 lb. margarine

1 lb. marshmallows

Melt above and add cracker crumbs. 3/4 c. grated raisins 1 tsp. coconut flavouring 1/2 c. dried apricots 1/2 c. raw cranberries 3/4 c. dates, cut up Add to first mixture and mix well. Pat mixture in 6"x13"x2" pan lined with plastic wrap. Chill.

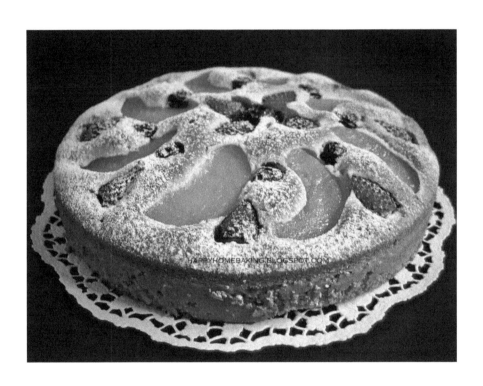

DIABETIC RAISIN CAKE

2 c. water
2 c. raisins

Cook until water evaporates. Add: 2 eggs 2 tbsp. sweetener 3/4 c. cooking oil 1 tsp. soda 2 c. flour 1 1/2 tsp. cinnamon 1 tsp. vanilla Mix well. Pour into 8"x8" greased pan, bake at 350 degrees for 2 minutes. Makes 20 servings. 1 fruit, 2 fat, 185 calories.

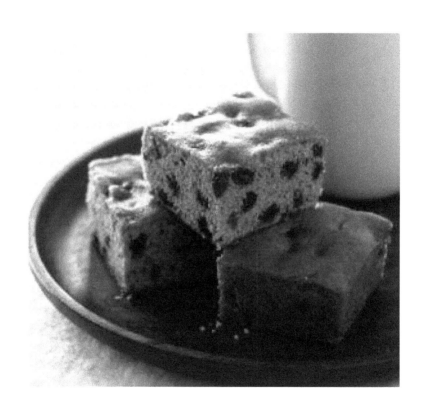

DIABETIC SPONGE CAKE

7 eggs

1/2 c. fruit juice, orange

3 tbsp. Sweet 'n Low or any sugar
substitute 2 tbsp. lemon juice

3/4 tsp. cream of tartar 1
1/2 c. sifted cake flour
1/4 tsp. salt

Separate eggs. Beat egg whites with salt until foamy. Add cream
of tartar and continue beating until stiff. In another bowl,
combine rest of ingredients and mix well. Fold in beaten egg
whites. Bake in greased and floured bundt pan at 350 degrees for
40 minutes or longer; test with toothpick. Serve with no sugar
jelly (all fruit) and Cool Whip.

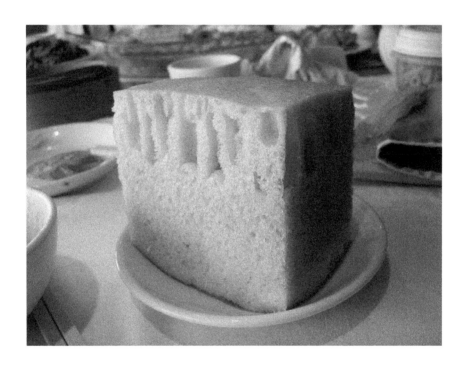

DIABETIC ORANGE DATE BARS

1 c. chopped dates 1/4
c. sugar

1/3 c. vegetable oil
1/2 c. orange juice 1
c. all-purpose flour

1/2 c. chopped pecans 1
egg

1 1/2 tsp. baking powder 1
tbsp. grated orange rind

Combine dates, sugar, oil and juice in a saucepan. Cook for 5
minutes to soften dates. Cool. Add remaining ingredients.
Spread into an oiled 8"x8" baking pan. Bake in 350-degree oven
for 25 to 30 minutes. Cool before cutting. Makes 36 bars.

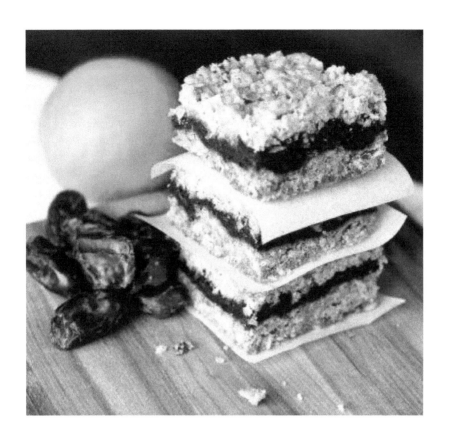

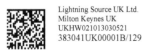
Lightning Source UK Ltd.
Milton Keynes UK
UKHW021013030521
383041UK00001B/129